# My A-Z
# (Myalgic Ence

## Fifty poems about living with Myalgic Encephalomyelitis

By
Ros Lemarchand

© 2013 Ros Lemarchand

**I dedicate this book to all those living with chronic and invisible illness**

# Foreword

This special collection of poems will undoubtedly resonate with anyone facing the challenge of chronic illness and will also be easily accessible for friends, family, or anyone with a willingness to understand myalgic encephalomyelitis (ME). These poems represent what it can be like to live on a daily basis, year to year, often decade to decade, with an illness like myalgic encephalomyelitis. There are such a number and variety of effects and symptoms that can fluctuate markedly from day to day and even hour to hour or moment to moment.

Ros Lemarchand writes from her own experiences and feelings as well as those of others as expressed on social networking sites and other internet forums. These sites can be a lifeline for people who are housebound due to chronic or disabling illness. With a professional background in education, a range of life experiences, insight, common sense, compassion, warmth and humour, Ros plays an important and highly valued role in providing help and support to others through this medium, whilst coping with her own challenges in battling this chronic illness.

ME is a complex disease, usually triggered by the immune system, but with effects on potentially every system and organ of the body. The severity can range from mild to very severe and can fluctuate in the same person over time. It can remain the same, gradually improve or even worsen. Mild ME is defined by experts as a 50% loss of function. Most people might imagine what impact that would have on their life. At its most severe, people with ME may be confined to lie in quiet, darkened rooms because of painful sensitivity to light, sound and touch. They may be unable to self-care, may have partial or full paralysis, seizures and may need feeding by tube.

Like many other diseases, ME has been called different names over the years. Some well known figures from history had ME-like chronic illness, including Charles Darwin and Florence

Nightingale, whose birthday was chosen for an international day of awareness on May 12th. Over 60 outbreaks have been recorded worldwide since 1934. It was first defined as myalgic encephalomyelitis by Dr. Melvin Ramsay after one such outbreak at The Royal Free Hospital in London in 1955. The World Health Organisation (WHO) classified it as a neurological disease in 1969 (WHO ICD-10 G93.3) along with post-viral fatigue syndrome. In the late 1980s, the American Centres for Disease Control (CDC) were called upon to investigate outbreaks of an ME-like illness, which they decided to name chronic fatigue syndrome (CFS). This is easily confused with fatigue syndrome, which is classified by WHO under Mental Health and so this led medical professionals the world over to treat CFS, and thus ME and PVFS, as somatoform disorders – physical symptoms with psychological cause. Other words with the same meaning are psychosomatic, non-organic, functional and factitious. Estimates of full recovery from the original Ramsay-defined ME are less than 10%, so this lack of understanding causes untold suffering.

A percentage from the sale of this book will be donated to the charity Invest in ME (IiME). Established in 2006, IiME educate and campaign for change in the way that ME is perceived and treated by governments, media and the medical profession, while also supporting individuals and families. They support, organise and fund 1st class scientific research to find diagnostic tests and effective medical treatment options for ME.

Ros's creative flair, complemented by the artwork of fellow sufferers, will be a book to treasure for its poetic artistry and in the hope that one day soon, thanks to IiME and their supporters, it may also have a place in the archives of medical history.

Jo Best
Invest in ME
www.investinme.org
Let's do it for ME!
http://ldifme.org

## With thanks to the following

I would like to thank Rob Wilson for creating the front and back cover of this book.

Thank you to Jo Best for her help and support, and for all the campaigning and awareness raising that she does despite her health problems.

Thank you to Julia Cottam who gave me the encouragement as well as help and support to share my poems.

Thank you to my husband Didier and daughter who have helped and supported me from the beginning of my illness.

Thank you to my long standing and faithful friends Cathy, Teresa and Di who have always been there for me.

Thank you for all the wonderful friends I have found on social network sites. You have been a wonderful help and support. I couldn't have done all this without you.

Finally I would like to thank my parents who gave me a love of poetry.

# Introduction

I first became ill in 2002 and at the time I didn't know what was wrong with me. It felt like the worst flu ever but it didn't go away. I tried courageously many times to carry on working until I completely collapsed. My doctor at the time hadn't got a clue. So I changed doctors, was sent for lots of tests and by a process of elimination I was told in 2003 that I had chronic fatigue syndrome. Although it was a relief to have a name to my illness I knew nothing about it. So I read as much as I could in order to learn more. I soon discovered the original name was myalgic encephalomyelitis and I now prefer to use that name whenever possible. Chronic fatigue syndrome just sounds like I'm a bit tired and it's so much more than that.

Since my diagnosis I have struggled with a very difficult and invisible illness. I have faced disbelief and ignorance from family, friends, doctors and many others. I still do to this day. Many people with M.E. or other chronic and invisible illnesses share the same experiences.
I had to stop working and consider my health. I was suffering on many fronts and was only getting worse not better. It was a hard decision to make. So my life had to change. At times it's made me feel angry, frustrated or even depressed. I have gone through a grieving process. I've lost that person I once used to be. I've lost the life I once had. I have been forced to change, adapt and learn ways of coping with a chronic illness.

As M.E. is a remitting and relapsing illness I've had good periods and some really bad ones. It's an illness forever changing and new symptoms developing all the time. With little or no support from the medical profession I've had to learn about this illness and how best to manage it myself. Over the years I have probably become a self expert. Yet even now this illness can still take me by surprise.

Fortunately I have found help and support from others like myself on social networking sites and other internet forums. Without this support I don't know how I would have survived. It's comforting and reassuring to know that I am not facing this alone. I have observed others expressing the same feelings, emotions, experiences and problems as myself. This has given me the inspiration for many of my poems.

Through my poems I have been able to express not only how I feel but others as well. My poems are a window on what it's like to live with M.E., how it affects and changes lives, the suffering with so many symptoms, the lack of understanding, the emotions and experiences that so many have in common.

This book is a collection of my poems that I have written over a number of years. Writing poems has helped me to cope with this very difficult illness. I hope that by sharing my poems in this book it helps others to do the same. My poems are primarily about M.E. but I'm sure they can apply to other chronic or invisible illnesses.

If you have been diagnosed with M.E., or even another invisible illness, I hope you will be able to identify with my poems. If you don't have M.E. I hope that my poems help you to understand this difficult and complex illness. I hope that it will help you to gain some small insight to what it's like to live with M.E. Through my poems I want to show the reality of a life with M.E. and to increase understanding and awareness. And that's why a percentage of this book will go to the UK Charity Invest in M.E. (IiME) who do so much for the cause of M.E. in raising awareness and understanding.
Thank you
Ros Lemarchand

## My A-Z of M.E.

ANGRY since I feel my life has all gone
BORED as endless days go on and on
CRYING when no one can understand me
DEPRESSED because of this illness M.E.
EXHAUSTED after every effort I make
FRUSTRATED by those who believe I'm a fake
GRIEVING for everything that I have lost
HAPPY to find new friendship at no cost
ISOLATED from a world that used to be mine
JEALOUS of those who can have a good time
KINDNESS from others who suffer the same
LOSS of so much and looking for blame
MISERABLE with no ending that is in sight
NIGHTMARES strange and real that give me a fright
OPTIMISTIC one day someone will find a cure
PAIN is strong and so hard to endure
QUESTIONS so many that have no answer
REST and rest hoping to feel better
SENSITIVE to so many things around me
TERRIFIED by symptoms that people can't see
UNDERSTANDING why is it so hard to explain?
VALUE my life though nothing is the same
WORRY because my body feels so weak
XRMV could this be the clue we seek?
YEARN to be healthy and to have some fun
ZOMBIE instead this is what I've become!

## Acceptance

To say "this illness I accept"
Is such a very hard concept
To accept my life has to change
To accept it can't stay the same
To accept how I must now live
To try not to be negative
To accept my limitations
To lower my expectations
To accept I need to take care
To accept energy is rare
To accept I need to have rest
To pace myself and do what's best
To accept new ways of coping
To find better understanding
To not be demanding on me
To reject those feelings guilty
To accept help on a bad day
To be honest in what I say
To accept I'll have some bad days
And to feel denial and rage
To stop fighting against my fate
To stop my anger and my hate
To again find myself grieving
To mourn that life I'm now missing
To accept does not mean defeat
To know this illness I will beat
To accept is not giving in
But hope one day this fight I'll win
To accept part goes to M.E.
To know it can't take the real me!
I wish I could say "I accept"
But it is such a hard concept.

## Alive but not living

Alive but not living
My life has lost meaning
I feel like I`m dreaming
And want to start screaming
I think of life missing
And go into grieving
There comes some accepting
Yet I can`t help crying
Part of me is changing
There is no denying
For sure I`m not lying
Believe me I`m trying
So hard to keep breathing
Carry on believing
Not to give up hoping
For a cure I`m praying
How I hate this feeling
It`s all so frustrating
I try to keep smiling
But it`s so depressing
Survive but not living
So tired of fighting
Feel no one is helping
I`m left slowly dying.

## Angry

I hate you
Look what you`ve done!
My life is gone.

I hate you
Making me sick
So very quick

I hate you
Please go away
Why do you stay?

I hate you
You`ve cheated me
Of all that`s me

I hate you
Here all the time
Wrecked life of mine

I hate you
Give me a break
From pain and ache!

I hate you
For ending dreams
No hope it seems

I hate you
And my life now
But accept how?

I hate you
You make me sad
You make me mad!

I hate you
I cry and shout
Just go, get out!

I hate you
You make me cry
And I ask why?

I hate you
Poison in me
Known as M.E.

**BORED**

Bored as endless days go on and on
Bored by mindless days with the tv on
Bored and pointless days which I try to fill
Bored and hopeless days when I feel ill
Bored when sleepless nights just past so slow
Bored by aimless weeks with nought to show
Bored as endless days go on and on

**BORED**

## Brain Fog

My head feels light
Doesn't seem right
Can't think at all
Hard to recall
Lost words I seek
When want to speak
Then say wrong words
That sound absurd
Confuse a name
Brain fog to blame
Often forget
Then get upset
It's hard to spell
Or write so well
Make notes to aid
For actions made
Weird sensation
Much frustration
Feels so scary
Makes me wary
Memory lost
But at what cost?
I feel so blank
M.E. to thank!

## Crazy

I suspect I`m going crazy
As no one seems to believe me!
All say that I look so healthy
Since there is nothing they can see.

I feel that I`m going crazy
As I have such a strange feeling.
Some say I`m idle and lazy
But they have no understanding.

I think that maybe I`m crazy
And perhaps it`s all in my head
I used to be very healthy
But now I`m disabled instead.

I wonder if I`ve gone crazy
Or maybe it`s all a bad dream
Then I`ll wake to reality
And things are truly as they seem.

Is it my imagination?
Am I really losing my mind?
There must be some explanation
If only the cause I could find.

My self doubt is now growing strong
As all say that I look "just fine"
Perhaps I have got this all wrong
For there is no obvious sign.

"Snap out of it" people tell me
If only it was that easy.
I have invisible M.E.
Which is so difficult to see.

This is such a crazy illness
I know I`m not losing my mind
But all the doubt is causing stress
While there is nothing wrong to find!

**Crying**

I have a cry today
As memories revive
Of life that's gone away
And how I just survive

My angry tears do fall
It's really so unfair
Injustice of it all
Right now too hard to bare.

I cry with frustration
When the words elude me
It's a degradation
Of my ability

I find myself crying
When I try to explain
There's no understanding
Of how much I'm in pain

Today I start crying
I'm fed up with life now
Why should I keep trying?
What's the point anyhow?

I have a cry today
This is no life for me
Sick of feeling this way
Because of my M.E.!

**Dead but still breathing!**

I`m dead but still breathing
Frozen and cold
It`s a dreadful feeling
That`s taken hold.
Not awake or dreaming
But paralyzed
"Help me" I try screaming
So terrified.
I feel like I`m dying
My heart is weak
It`s hard to be moving
To think or speak.
My body is struggling
Feel I can`t breathe
Makes me anxious and scared
When will it ease?
It`s all so frightening
If I`m alone
I can`t help panicking
Who can I phone?
I feel dead yet living
Poison in me
There must be an ending
To set me free!

### **Depressed**

**D**ead but I'm still living
**E**mpty of all meaning
**P**ointless just existing
**R**eason is now fading
**E**ndless days of drifting
**S**ad my past life grieving
**S**ad and feel like crying
**E**nd my life I'm thinking
**D**eath is more appealing.

## Don't

Don't assume because I'm younger than you
I'm healthy, strong and can stand in this queue.
Don't think I have plenty of energy
At seventy-five you have more than me!
Don't look at me as if I have no right
The last thing I want is to make a fight.
Don't say that there is nothing wrong with me
My handicap is not easy to see.
Don't be so rude, please show me some respect
It's what I deserve and hope to expect.
Don't treat me like a liar and a fake
This illness is for real, make no mistake!
Don't be so cruel and cause me distress
When you say it's nothing but laziness.
Don't judge me when you don't understand
I'm truly ill and need a lending hand.
Don't tell me how I really look so well
It's only those closest to me can tell.
Don't you consider how hurt I might be
By your words and actions made carelessly.
Don't assume that you have priority
I have proof of my disability!

# Emotions of M.E.

### Angry
When I'm treated like a fake
Is it worth the energy to educate?

### Hurt
By many a cruel comment
You've no idea of my pain and torment

### Fed up
Of those who can't understand
Think I am well and don't need a helping hand

### Sad
I've lost family and friend
Because this illness they cannot comprehend

### Lonely
Most days I spend all alone
No person I see or speak to on the phone

### Disappointed
Not to make that planned trip out
Leaves me feeling like I want to cry or shout

### Upset
When I'm confined to my bed
But I need to rest my sick body and head

### Hate
Having no control in life
How can I plan to do anything I like?

### Grieved
I feel my life has ended
So much lost with no chance it can be mended

### Depressed
As there`s no ending in sight
Hard to continue this unrelenting fight

### Stressed
By benefit I must claim
But how difficult I find it to explain

### Scared
When I can`t breathe properly
Feels like my life is slipping away from me

### Frightened
By nightmares or a strange dream
That seem so real and lifelike, what do they mean?

### Anxious
And panic with any stress
Which makes my symptoms worse and causes distress

### Annoyed
When I can`t recall a word
I feel brain dead, confused and somewhat absurd!

### Distraught
So many tears with this pain
All I want is to feel normal once again?

**Frustration**
By the ignorance I find
From doctors with no answer and doubt of mind

**Despair**
After all kinds of treatment
I'm thinking there's no cure apart from heaven sent

**Exasperated**
When sleep eludes me each night
Even though I'm exhausted and need respite

**Irritation**
When you say I look so well
But I feel so very ill. Why you can't tell?

**Happy**
When I have a better day
To feel maybe this illness will go away

**Exhausted**

I hit a wall of exhaustion
Unable to do any more
Like a huge wave without warning
Suddenly I crash to the floor

It`s like someone has cut my strings
I can no longer stand or walk
My body is weak and shaking
My mind is blank and I can`t talk

I`m trying hard not to panic
By this loss of my energy
But I can barely move or breathe
And it all seems rather scary

I feel nauseous and sweaty
Like my life is draining from me
It`s hard to describe this feeling
Compares to a dead battery

I rest and wait to feel better
Maybe I should have a sleep now
Yet even though I`m exhausted
Any sleep eludes me somehow

**Fear**
That no one can understand me
Hide the truth or I'll seem crazy
**Fear**
To pay my doctor a visit
He may say there's nothing in it!
**Fear**
Of all the tests I'll have to make
Results making me look a fake
**Fear**
I'll be asked to do CBT
Say I'm depressed or unhappy
**Fear**
That I'll be forced to follow GET
And all of their demands be met
**Fear**
I'll be left totally alone
With no help, to cope on my own
**Fear**
Of a future that now looks bleak
What can I do feeling so weak?
**Fear**
That my life has come to an end
A prayer to God I must now send!


***CBT*** *is cognitive behaviour therapy and is a way of talking about how you think about yourself, the world and other people and how what you do affects your thoughts and feelings.*

***GET*** *is graded exercise therapy is physical activity that starts very slowly and gradually increases over time. This approach is used as part of a treatment plan for chronic fatigue syndrome (CFS) and certain other conditions*

You make me
**Frustrated**
So angry
And irritated

You make me
**Frustrated**
So tearful
And feel defeated

You make me
**Frustrated**
Uncertain
And disappointed

You make me
**Frustrated**
A failure
And my life`s wasted

You make me
**Frustrated**
Cry and shout
That you are hated

Get out!

## Grieving

It`s a bad case of flu
I`m sure I`ll recover
In just a week or two
Then it will be over

I`ll push through this feeling
There`s nothing wrong with me
I`ll soon start to healing
And feel fine and healthy

I hate feeling like this
What`s happening to me?
I know something`s amiss
I`m running on empty

I can`t go on the same
But I don`t want to stop
Something will have to change
Otherwise I`ll soon drop

I refuse to accept
There`s something wrong with me
Many tears I have wept
Frustrated and angry

Perhaps if I rest more
Or stay in bed all day
I`ll get back as before
And this will go away

It`s all so frustrating
Despite all that I`ve done
I feel like I`m sinking
And my life has all gone

I want my old life back
This really is not fair
At work I got the sack
And I can`t go back there

Now there`s uncertainty
In the future for me
Must face reality
A new life with M.E.

It`s all so depressing
I`ve lost what once was me
And all that I`m dreaming
Now taken by M.E.

I think this is my fate
So trying to accept
And let go of my hate
But it`s a hard concept

I`m coming to terms now
With a new life for me
I`ve no choice anyhow
But to live with M.E.

## Happy

I used to be happy
Look forward to each day
Then M.E. came along
And took it all away!

My happiness was gone
Replaced by a grieving
Anger and frustration
And numb kind of feeling.

I thought life had ended
And chance for happiness
With all my days now filled
By this chronic illness

Yet slowly there has been
Acceptance within me
Adjustment of my life
New ways to be happy.

**Hope**
To have a better day
The pain to go away
**Hope**
This fatigue will soon end
And my body can mend
**Hope**
To find energy
Then start recovery
**Hope**
To improve my pacing
Against all I'm facing
**Hope**
I find new ways to cope
Which come within my scope
**Hope**
To increase more awareness
So disbelief is less
**Hope**
That I can work again
And all's not lost in vain
**Hope**
To better understand
This dreadful M.E. land
**Hope**
For a future healthy
And at last M.E. free!

## Hot and Cold

My thermostat
Is not working
Out of control
Either too hot
Or very cold!
How can I be
Both hot and cold?
Body confused
Instead chaos
Has taken hold!
Don`t understand
Why I feel hot
When it is cold
Why I feel cold
When it is hot!
Temperature
Always changing
Never the same
One minute cold
And then BOILING!
A sudden sweat
Comes over me
Take off layers
But then I feel
Cold instantly!
Hard to control
And keep stable
What must I do
To make myself
Comfortable?

**I am visible**

I am visible
Oh why can't you see
My illness and me?

Oh why don't you look
And see in my eyes
I'm telling no lies?

Why don't you believe
That I'm truly sick
And this is no trick?

Oh why don't you see
This is not a show?
You don't want to know!

Why don't you notice
That I'm not the same?
Illness is to blame.

Why can't you discern
The changes in me?
Surely you can see!

Oh why can't you sense
My pain, my distress
And unhappiness?

Oh why can't you see
I've no energy?
That's too much for me!

Why do you ignore
The way I'm feeling?
The truth concealing!

So why don't you ask
How I really feel?
My illness is real!

Oh why can't you see
What is wrong with me?
Where's your sympathy?

Why do you avoid
Talking to my face?
Try taking my place!

Why don't you listen?
Do I have to scream
So that I'll be seen?

Why do you pretend
I'm not really there?
That's cruel and unfair!

Why can't you accept,
Though it's hard to see,
Disability?

It is visible
If only you'd see
This illness and me!

## I Look Back

I look back
And what do I see?
Someone else
That I used to be,
A person
Happy and carefree,
A life that
Was full and busy,
A purpose
With some dreams for me,
A stranger
Was that really me?
Look forward
And what do I see?
I'm not sure
What I can now be,
All is lost
A life that's empty,
Life ended
No future for me,
A new life
I must make for me,
A life sick
A life with M.E.

**Isolated**
From all I know
From all I love
Fills me with woe

**Isolated**
From family
Don`t understand
Or visit me

**Isolated**
As friends I lose
Living alone
Now a recluse

**Isolated**
New friends `online`
Virtual world
Eases my time

**Isolated**
Sick and in pain
My life now changed
Nothing the same

**Isolated**
And so lonely
I cry some tears
Thinking "If only"

**Isolated**
Each endless day
In these four walls
I have to stay

**Isolated**
I hope and pray
I can escape
And get away

**Isoated**
Watching outside
Through my window
Life that`s not mine

**Isolated**
Behind a veil
Trapped inside
Just like a jail

**Jealous**
Of those who can have a good time
Reminds me of a life once mine

**Jealous**
Of those who are healthy and fit
That was me until I lost it

**Jealous**
Of those who go to work each day
I never thought I'd feel that way

**Jealous**
Of those who can plan life ahead
Mine is wrecked and I stay in bed

**Jealous**
Of those who can fulfil their dreams
Now my life has ended it seems

## Kindness

The kindness of others
Who all suffer the same
Provides me with support
And helps to keep me sane!

When I read your kind words
Tears well up in my eyes
It`s so overwhelming
Taking me by surprise

Such a little kindness
I find goes a long way
And makes a difference
To a difficult day

A few kind words and thoughts
I sure appreciate
And I thank you so much
My friends are truly great.

**Loss**

I've lost so much
The life I knew
Illness to blame
Must start anew

I've lost my job
And career too
No hope for me
What can I do?

Now my lifestyle
Can't stay the same
With no money
It has to change

My house is sold
I'll have no home
So where to go?
As yet unknown

Soon to lose my
Security
Which then causes
Anxiety

Family and friends
All stay away
Don't understand
Or what to say

Loss of freedom
To go outside
Home a prison
Where I now hide

My social life
Does not exist
So many names
Crossed off my list

As for hobbies
I can't pursue
All pleasure lost
In what I do

No longer have
The energy
Or cognitive
Ability

No stamina
Get up and go
No endurance
Or libido!

I've lost control
Of my body
All function gone
Such a worry

Memory loss
The wrong words used
Names forgotten
Or they're confused

Concentration
Hard to maintain
Brain fog blocks me
And clouds the brain

Loss of balance
With dizzy head
So hard to walk
Prefer my bed

Loss of some weight
And appetite
Feel sick and weak
Stomach not right

I`ve lost all hope
And what I dream
My purpose gone
With self esteem

I`ve lost my faith
In so much now
I want to pray
But don`t know how

I`ve lost my life
The will to live
Feels like the end
No more to give

## M.E. Groundhog Day

On this International M.E. Day
All my symptoms are very much the same.
And I feel like it's M.E. Groundhog Day
As the pattern repeats over again.

On this International M.E. Day
I am still hoping to get my life back.
But it seems this illness is here to stay
And I can't return to a healthy track.

On this International M.E. Day
I'm still waiting for that magical cure
I read and follow what scientists say
As yet nothing is definite or sure.

On this International M.E. Day
There is no certain guaranteed treatment.
I've tried everything that's come my way
But it only leads to disappointment.

On this International M.E. Day
There are still many who don't believe me.
So raising awareness should help today
With understanding and more clarity

On this International M.E. Day
I want to share how I and others feel.
We are all waiting for a better day
And acceptance that this illness is real.

On this International M.E. Day
I wish I'd more positive news to say.
I long for this illness to go away.
Instead it's back to M.E. Groundhog Day!

**May 12th is International M.E./CFS & FM Awareness Day.**
May 12 was chosen as it coincided with the birth date of Florence Nightingale, the English army nurse who inspired the founding of the International Red Cross. Nightingale became chronically ill in her mid-thirties with a Myalgic Encephalomyelitis/Chronic Fatigue Syndrome (ME/CFS)-like illness.
I called this poem M.E. Groundhog Day after the film of that name where the same day is repeated over and over again. M.E. is much like that. And like in the film we are forced to reexamine our lives and priorities because of this illness.
http://www.may12th.org/

## M.E. Sleep patterns

At first I slept
All day and night
Always tired
Not feeling right

I slept so much
Yet still felt bad
It was as if
No sleep I'd had

I couldn't wake
In the morning
But felt alert
By the evening

My sleep became
More disrupted
Which dreams or pain
Interrupted

My sleep pattern
Started to change
Insomnia
Taking the stage

Impossible
To sleep all night
Wake unrefreshed
By the daylight

Even though I
Feel so tired
I cannot sleep
And feel wired

So many nights
I lie awake
But how to sleep
What does it take?

A good night`s sleep
I need to heal
And then maybe
Better I`ll feel

## Miserable

Miserable with no ending in sight
I no longer want to keep up the fight

Now my life has lost all of its meaning
And with it my hope for plans I'm dreaming

How can I go on yet another day?
If I had faith perhaps then I could pray

Nothing seems to have changed with the years past
And I feel my life is declining fast

Miserable and sorry for myself
As if the world has left me on a shelf

Miserable with no ending in sight
But perhaps tomorrow I'll feel alright!

## My bed

I love my bed
I hate my bed
I live in my bed
I sleep in my bed
I wake in my bed
I rest in my bed
I eat in my bed
I drink in my bed
I think in my bed
I read in my bed
I write in my bed
I dream in my bed
I hurt in my bed
I`m hot in my bed
I sweat in my bed
I`m cold in my bed
I`m sick in my bed
I cry in my bed
I scream in my bed
I can`t leave my bed
I`m stuck in my bed
I hibernate in my bed
I take comfort in my bed
I`m paralysed in my bed
I watch the world from my bed
Now I want to leave my bed
I`ve been so long in my bed
Perhaps I`ll die in my bed

**Nightmares and dreams**

Nightmares
Strange and real
They give me
Such a fright
As they`re scary

Weird dreams
Are disturbed
And wake me
So confuse
Reality

Some dreams
Take hold and
I lose track
Of what`s real
And can`t get back

Long dreams
Seem to last
All the night
Repeating
Until daylight

Strange dreams
So vivid
Disturb me
Take over
My world nightly

Bad dreams
That upset
And make me
Start crying
Surprisingly

Nightmares
Unsettle
And shake me
Or sometimes
Paralyse me

Nightmares
And my dreams
Disrupt me
Most nights so
I sleep badly!

## Normal

Normal
What does that mean?
To me it's only in a dream

To sleep
The whole night through
Four hours is the best I can do

At work
Five days a week
Of that I can no longer speak

Career
This started well
Now it's all shot and gone to hell!

Shopping
A happy event
Perhaps an exhausting hour spent

The pub
A beer or two
But alcohol is now taboo!

Visit
My family
Is always difficult for me

Talking
On phone with friends
With mental fatigue it soon ends

A walk
What a pleasure
Hundred metres is my measure

Bike ride
Down country road
Instead my bike is better sold

Romance
And chance for love
Instead I look to heaven above

Marriage
One of my dreams
Now that is unlikely it seems

Children
A hope one day
What chance now I am forced to say

Normal
What does that mean?
Hope lost, life wrecked, a broken dream.............!!!

**Optimistic**

One day
Some one
Will find
A cure
And I
Will be
Healthy
Once more

So hard
To be
As years
Go past
To hope
That I`ll
Be well
At last!

## Pain

Pain in my head
Face or eyes
Throat and glands
Enlarged in size
Pain in my neck
And shoulder
That makes me
Feel much older
Pain in my ribs
And my thighs
That takes me
By some surprise
Pain in my wrists
And each hand
Hard to grasp
Or understand
Pain in my legs
And in my knees
New to me
How to relieve?
Pain in my feet
And my toes
Even down
To both my soles!
Pain in my bones
All way through
It`s so hard
What can I do?

Pain that
Is strong
And so
Hard to
Endure
So much pain
Awful pain
Chronic pain
Severe pain
Widespread pain
Terrible pain
Horrendous pain
Persistent pain
Unexplained pain
Disabling pain
Terrifying pain
Radiating pain
Unrelenting pain
Unbearable pain
Agonising pain
Excruciating Pain!
**Pain!!!!!!!!!!!!!!!**

## Pyjamas

A life in pyjamas
I have no choice to stay
I'm too ill for a wash
Or change on any day

I love my pyjamas
They're so cosy and warm
My clothes are forgotten
All fading and unworn

I live in pyjamas
It's all that I need now
I never go outside
And leave home anyhow

I stay in pyjamas
No energy to dress
My hair is all matted
And I look such a mess

I look for pyjamas
That are cute and funny
They replace my real clothes
And save lots of money

I life in pyjamas
Feeling so ill each day
Unable to get dressed
So this is how I'll stay!

## Questions

Why me?
Why now?
M.E.?
But how?

Will I die?
Is this it?
Please don't lie
Just fix it!

What is M.E.?
What is to blame?
It's new to me
Don't feel the same

Am I dreaming?
This can't be real
I'm still breathing
Yet dead I feel

How long will it last?
Will I recover?
I hope it ends fast
Or my life's over

How can you help me?
What is the treatment?
GET and CBT
Is all you present

What else can you tell me?
I need to learn much more
Of this illness M.E.
And what I have in store.

**Rest**

    Rest
    Rest
    Rest
And hope to get better
That`s my advice to you
You know it makes sense as
It`s the best thing to do

    Rest
    Rest
    Rest
And hope to feel better
I know it`s hard to do
But it`s the only thing
That will benefit you

    Rest
    Rest
    Rest
Listen to what I say
Your body needs to heal
And have a proper rest
As exhausted you feel

    Rest
    Rest
    Rest
Let your mind become still
Repose your tired brain
Clear away all your thoughts
As they are only a drain

Rest
Rest
Rest
Stop! It`s now time to rest
This is the remedy
When you are in relapse
Towards recovery!

**Scream**

I want to
Scream
And
Shout
I need to
Let
It
Out
I want to
Cry
And
Yell
I have to
Leave
This
Hell
I want to
Swear
And
Kick
I don`t want
To
Be
Sick!

## Sensitive

Sensitive to
So many things
Around me

Sensitive to
So much noise that
Surrounds me

Sensitive to
Any bright light
Which blinds me

Sensitive to
Many smells that
Confront me

Sensitive to
Food I eat which
Upsets me

Sensitive to
Many drugs that
Should help me

Sensitive to
Chemicals that
Affect me

Sensitive to
Any stress that
Panics me

Sensitive to
So much and tears
Come quickly

Sensitive to
So many things
Around me

So I want to
Hibernate and
Protect me!

# Sleep

My bed to sleep
But stay awake
Why can`t I sleep?
For goodness sake!

Finally sleep
Then wake at one.
Call that a sleep?
It`s far from done!

Drift off to sleep
Yet wake at two!
Need longer sleep
What can I do?

Again I sleep
But wake at three
If I can`t sleep
Should I make tea?

Eyes shut once more
A dream wakes me
It`s only four
Too dark to see!

I lie awake
And start thinking
That`s a mistake
Stops me sleeping!

What time is it?
Must sleep somehow
I don`t believe it
Only five now!

It`s six at last
And I`m not sure
Early Breakfast
Or sleep once more?

Chink of day light
The sign of dawn
Oh what a night
Give a big yawn!

So exhausted
Through lack of sleep
And frustrated
I need some sleep!

## Terrified

Terrified by symptoms
That people can't see
Who think that I'm faking
And don't believe me

Terrified when I breathe
By pains in my chest
I feel like I'm dying
Must lay down to rest

Terrified I might fall
With this dizziness
The loss of my balance
And light-headedness

Terrified that I will
Remain paralysed
In my arms or my legs
Like I'm petrified

Terrified when I can't
Think or concentrate
And I forget so much
Which I really hate

Terrified I'll be left
Totally alone
No family or friends
To cope on my own

Terrified I may hear
That my benefit
Is going to be stopped
And my life with it

Terrified I`ll be told
A job I must find
That I`m not really ill
It`s all in my mind

Terrified that I may
Lose my house and home
I`ll have nowhere to live
Lose all that I own

Terrified that I will
Never leave my bed
My life is at an end
And I`ll soon be dead

## Trapped

Inside this body I feel trapped
Hard to move and energy sapped.
A pain that keeps me in this shell
It's like my own personal hell.
Unable to open my eyes,
Get dressed or out of my bed rise.
Like a bubble, smaller each day,
I see my life slipping away.
Cut off and in my home I hide,
To relinquish that world outside.
Isolated from all I've known
Now living my life all alone.
It's like I've moved to M.E. land
A country hard to understand
No longer able to see me
That person I wanted to be.
This world is not of my choosing
And now there's so much I'm loosing
Friendships difficult to maintain
My illness too hard to explain
My family all stay away
Avoid me, unsure what to say.
I want to end this trapped feeling
And to find a way of healing.
I want to break free from this pain
So I can start living again.
I want to escape this purdah
I feel I can go no further!

## Understanding

Why is it
So hard to
Explain?
Why must I
Repeat once
Again?
Why can`t you
See that I`m
In pain?
Why can`t you
See what`s wrong
With me?
Why don`t you
Support and
Help me?
Why can`t you
Understand M.E.?

## Value

Now I value my life
Though nothing is the same
So much has been stolen
Yet here I still remain

How I value myself
This person deep inside
Although my life has changed
The real me is alive

Did I value my life
Before illness arrived?
I thought I was dying
But somehow I survived

Now I value my life
It's so precious to me
And I go on living
Despite having M.E.

## Vulnerable

I feel vulnerable
Open and exposed.
I feel emotional
and on overload.
I feel so defenceless,
bare and insecure.
I feel so powerless,
weakened and unsure.
I feel loss of control
in all around me.
I feel trapped in a hole,
anxious with worry.
I feel so exhausted
and with no reserve.
I feel energy sapped
and need to conserve.
I feel so neglected,
lonely and alone.
I feel unprotected
so stay in my home.
I feel vulnerable,
very close to tears.
I feel emotional
and panic with fears.
I feel so overwhelmed
Uncertain and raw
I feel lost and engulfed
Can`t take any more!

## Worry

Worry
Because
My body
Feels so weak
My throat is
Hurting and
It`s hard to speak

Worry
Because
My heart is
Beating fast
I can`t breathe
And believe
This is my last

Worry
Because
My head is
Spinning round
I could lose
Balance and
Fall to the ground

Worry
Because
I can`t sleep
In the night
Lay awake
And worry
Until daylight

Worry
In case
I become
Paralyzed
Unable
To move and
Feel terrified

Worry
Because
My income
Is shrinking
At the same
Time my debts
Are increasing

Worry
Because
My future
Is unsure
My illness
Seems lifelong
And there`s no cure!

# XRMV

Gave hope for me
Possible chance
For recovery

I could see at last
Some help and a
Cure arriving fast

Thought you were to blame
The reason why
I was not the same

But what did it mean?
The puzzle solved?
Or was it a dream?

Links found to M.E.
With this virus
And poison in me

But it was false hope
And a dead end
That felt like a joke

Now it looks quite dead
And so it seems
That I was misled

XRMV is a retrovirus that controversial research linked to chronic fatigue syndrome. The controversy dates back to 2009 when a possible connection was found between chronic fatigue syndrome and XRMV. However the studies made in 2009 could not be reproduced and validated. Some researchers believe that contamination was to blame.

http://en.wikipedia.org/wiki/Xenotropic_murine_leukemia_virus-related_virus

## Yearn

I yearn to
Be healthy
And to
Have some fun
Go outside
To breathe the
Fresh air
In the sun
I yearn to
Be healthy
And to
Have some fun
Meet my friends
To drink, chat
Laugh, joke
Walk or run
I yearn to
Be healthy
And to
Have some fun
A zombie
Instead this
Is what
I`ve become!

**You**

You suddenly came without warning
I didn't know your name
I couldn't get up in the morning
Nothing felt quite the same.

So I paid my doctor a visit
She said it could be flu
But the symptoms didn't really fit
Hell, what was I to do?

I went back to her in frustration
She had nothing to say
Surely there was an explanation!
Angry, I walked away.

I still needed to find an answer
What this illness could be
I asked to see a second doctor
Who would surely help me!

He said that lots of tests should be made
To find out what was wrong
So then I began to feel afraid
Of what might come along

The day came at last to hear the truth
I hoped to have your name
Although the doctors had no real proof
A diagnosis came!

Chronic fatigue syndrome they called you
As all the tests were clear
There was nothing the doctors could do
Then I let fall a tear

Graded exercise was suggested
I knew nothing at all
Those doctors at the time I trusted
It led to my downfall!

After years of pain and suffering
I know you very well
The treatment and cure I'm still hoping
To end this living hell!!

## Zombie

A zombie I've now become
No expression on my face
All feeling and purpose gone
No longer part of the human race!

16150185R00063

Printed in Great Britain
by Amazon